LOW FODMAP DIET COOKBOOK FOR WOMEN

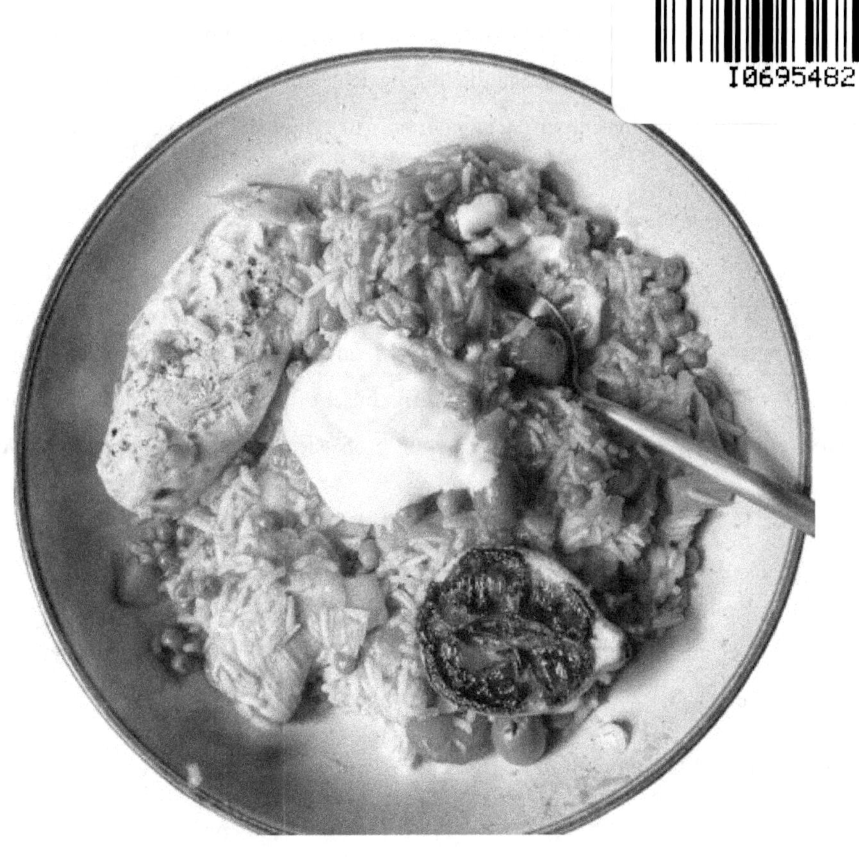

LYSANDRA QUINN

DISCLAIMER

The content within this book reflects my thoughts, experiences, and beliefs. It is meant for informational and entertainment purposes. While I have taken great care to provide accurate information, I cannot guarantee the absolute correctness or applicability of the content to every individual or situation. Please consult with relevant professionals for advice specific to your needs.

Contact the Author

Thank you for reading my book! I would love to hear from you, whether you have feedback, questions, or just want to share your thoughts. Your feedback means a lot to me and helps me improve as a writer.

Please don't hesitate to reach out to me through

contactmelysandraquinn@gmail.com

I look forward to connecting with my readers and appreciate your support in this literary journey. Your thoughts and comments are valuable to me.

TABLE OF CONTENTS

INTRODUCTION

In the quiet corners of culinary exploration, where the delicate balance of Flavors meets the intricacies of digestive health, I stumbled upon a journey that changed the life of my dear friend, Elaine. Hers was a tale of resilience, of countless attempts to find solace in the pages of various cookbooks that promised relief but delivered only frustration. Little did she know, as she navigated the labyrinth of dietary options, that the key to her well-being lay hidden in the heart of a Low FODMAP Diet.

Elaine, a vibrant soul encumbered by the relentless battles within her digestive system. She had traversed the realms of diets, each promising a remedy, yet none providing the sanctuary she so desperately sought. The culinary landscape was littered with failed attempts, leaving her disheartened and weary. It was in the midst of this gastronomic odyssey that I, a dedicated dietitian, decided to share the fruits of years spent researching and honing the art of Low FODMAP recipes.

As Elaine sceptically embarked on this culinary Endeavor, little did she anticipate the transformative power concealed within these carefully crafted recipes. A symphony of Flavors orchestrated to be gentle on her digestive system, each dish became a beacon of hope, dispelling the shadows that had long loomed over her well-being. It was a slow but steady ascent to vitality, and as the days turned into weeks, and weeks into months, Elaine found herself embracing a newfound sense of freedom.

And so, the seed of inspiration was planted. Witnessing the positive metamorphosis in Elaine's life, I felt an unwavering conviction to share this gift with women everywhere who, like Elaine, yearned for a culinary haven. Thus, the idea of this

Low FODMAP Diet Cookbook for Women was born—a collection of recipes that transcends the ordinary, designed not just for the body, but for the soul.

This cookbook is not merely a compilation of ingredients and instructions; it's a tapestry woven with care and compassion, a culinary guide that extends a comforting hand to women navigating the labyrinth of digestive distress. As a dietician, I understand the profound impact that food can have on one's well-being, and it is with this knowledge that I present to you a treasure trove of recipes that go beyond sustenance—they heal, nourish, and empower.

But before we delve into the heart of this cookbook, let me ask you a few questions:

- **Have you ever felt trapped in a cycle of dietary restrictions, desperately seeking a lifeline that would grant you the freedom to Savor the pleasures of food without the consequences?**
- **Do you, like Elaine, find yourself disheartened by the unfulfilled promises of countless cookbooks that claim to be the answer to your digestive woes?**
- **Can you recall the frustration of experimenting with recipes that left you feeling defeated, longing for a culinary companion that understands the intricacies of your body's unique needs?**

If your heart whispers 'yes' to any of these questions, then you're not alone. The journey to digestive well-being is a path often walked in solitude, and it is precisely for this reason that this cookbook extends its arms to embrace you. It's more than a collection of recipes; it's a testament to the possibility of a vibrant, fulfilling life fuelled by delicious meals that not only tantalize the taste buds but also nourish the body from within.

As we embark on this culinary voyage together, let the stories of women like Elaine serve as a beacon of hope. Within these pages, you will find not just recipes, but a narrative of resilience, a testament to the transformative power of a well-balanced, Low FODMAP diet. Each dish is a whisper of understanding, a gesture of solidarity with every woman yearning for a culinary haven in the face of digestive challenges.

Prepare to embark on a journey that transcends the realm of traditional cookbooks. Let the aromatic symphony of these recipes be the soundtrack to your triumph over digestive distress. As we turn the pages of this cookbook, may the stories within inspire you, the recipes delight you, and the journey ahead empower you to Savor not just the Flavors of life but the fullness of your well-being. Welcome to a world where the joy of eating is not just a pleasure but a healing ritual—a world crafted with love, dedication, and the heartfelt desire to see every woman thrive.

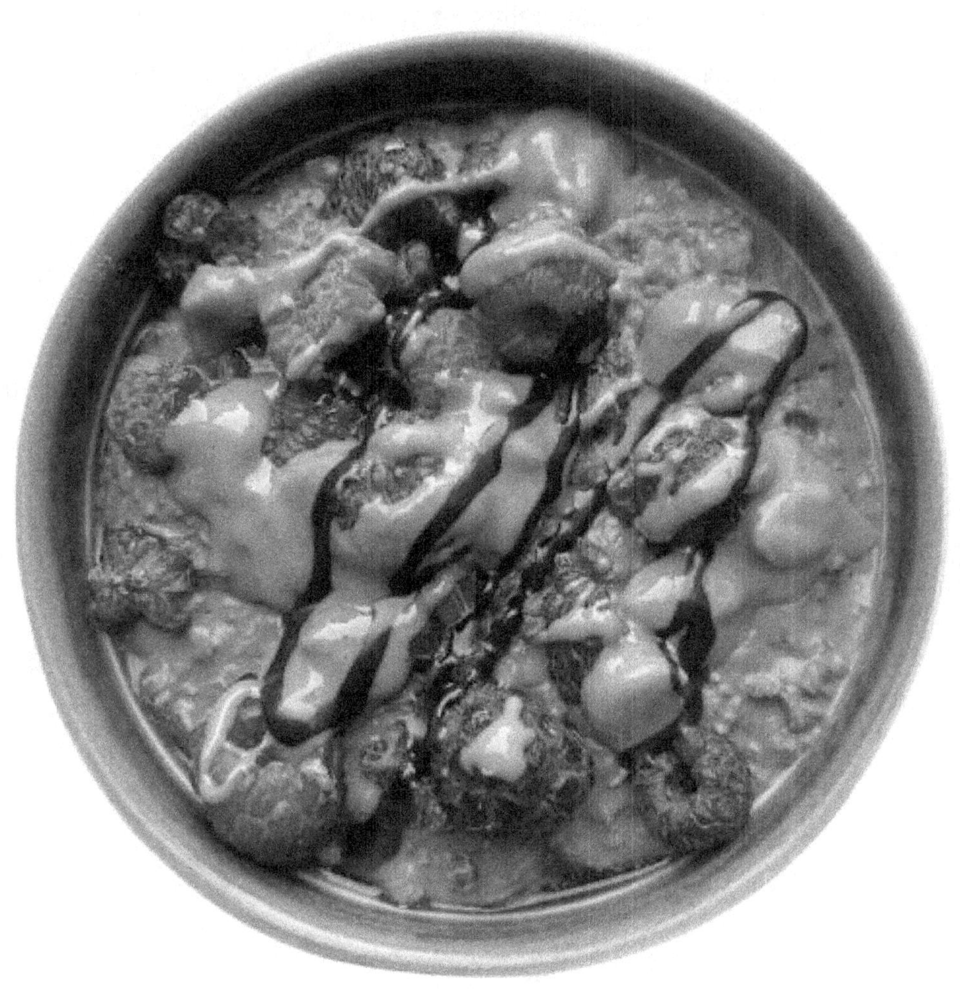

CHAPTER 1

WHAT ARE FODMAPS?

Fodmaps, which stands for Fermentable Oligosaccharides, Disaccharides, Monosaccharides, and Polyols, are a group of short-chain carbohydrates and sugar alcohols that are poorly absorbed in the small intestine. These substances are found in a variety of foods and include:

- Fermentable: They can be fermented by bacteria in the gut.
- Oligosaccharides: Found in some grains, vegetables, and fruits.
- Disaccharides: Include lactose, found in dairy products.
- Monosaccharides: Such as fructose, found in certain fruits.
- Polyols: Sugar alcohols found in certain fruits and vegetables, as well as used as artificial sweeteners.

How Fodmaps Can Affect Digestive Health

For some individuals, Fodmaps can trigger digestive symptoms such as bloating, gas, abdominal pain, and diarrhea. This is because these compounds draw water into the intestine and are fermented by bacteria in the gut, leading to the production of gas. In individuals with irritable bowel syndrome (IBS) or other functional gastrointestinal disorders, sensitivity to Fodmaps may exacerbate symptoms.

The digestion and absorption of Fodmaps can be incomplete, leading to these substances reaching the colon where they are fermented by bacteria. This fermentation process produces gases and can cause distension of the colon, contributing to symptoms in sensitive individuals.

Benefits of the Low FODMAP Diet for Women:

The Low FODMAP Diet has been found to be particularly beneficial for women, especially those dealing with digestive issues such as IBS. Some potential benefits include:

Symptom Relief: The primary aim of the Low FODMAP Diet is to alleviate symptoms associated with IBS, including bloating, gas, abdominal pain, and altered bowel habits.

Improved Quality of Life: By managing and reducing digestive symptoms, women may experience an improvement in their overall quality of life. The diet can help individuals regain control over their digestive health.

Individualized Approach: The Low FODMAP Diet is not a one-size-fits-all solution, and its success often relies on individualized adjustments. Women can work with healthcare professionals and dietitians to tailor the diet to their specific needs and preferences.

Identification of Trigger Foods: The diet involves an elimination phase followed by systematic reintroduction to identify specific Fodmaps that trigger symptoms. This personalized approach allows women to better understand their bodies and make informed dietary choices.

CHAPTER 2:

BREAKFAST DELIGHTS

Scrambled Eggs with Spinach and Feta:

Cooking Time: 10 minutes

Serving: 2

Ingredients:

- 4 large eggs
- 1 cup fresh spinach, chopped
- 1/4 cup crumbled feta cheese

Instructions:

1. Whisk eggs in a bowl.
2. Cook spinach in a non-stick pan until wilted.
3. Pour whisked eggs over spinach, scramble until cooked.
4. Sprinkle feta on top and serve.

Nutritional Information: (per serving)

Calories: 220, Protein: 16g, Fat: 15g, Carbohydrates: 4g

Greek Yogurt Parfait:

Cooking Time: 5 minutes

Serving: 1

Ingredients:

- 1 cup lactose-free Greek yogurt
- 1/2 cup blueberries
- 1 tablespoon chia seeds

Instructions:

1. Layer yogurt, blueberries, and chia seeds in a glass.
2. Repeat layers.
3. Top with a few extra blueberries.

Nutritional Information: (per serving)

Calories: 280, Protein: 20g, Fat: 10g, Carbohydrates: 25g

Quinoa Breakfast Bowl:

Cooking Time: 15 minutes

Serving: 2

Ingredients:

- 1 cup cooked quinoa
- 1/2 cup strawberries, sliced.
- 1 tablespoon pumpkin seeds

Instructions:

1. Mix quinoa, strawberries, and pumpkin seeds in a bowl.
2. Serve warm or cold.

Nutritional Information: (per serving)

Calories: 220, Protein: 8g, Fat: 6g, Carbohydrates: 35g

Smoked Salmon and Avocado Wrap:

Cooking Time: 10 minutes

Serving: 1

Ingredients:

- 1 gluten-free wrap
- 2 oz smoked salmon
- 1/2 avocado, sliced.

Instructions:

1. Place smoked salmon and avocado on the wrap.
2. Roll and slice in half.

Nutritional Information: (per serving)

Calories: 320, Protein: 20g, Fat: 18g, Carbohydrates: 25g

Banana and Almond Smoothie:

Cooking Time: 5 minutes

Serving: 1

Ingredients:

- 1 ripe banana
- 1 cup almond milk
- 1 tablespoon almond butter

Instructions:

1. Blend banana, almond milk, and almond butter until smooth.
2. Pour into a glass and enjoy.

Nutritional Information: (per serving)

Calories: 250, Protein: 5g, Fat: 12g, Carbohydrates: 30g

Spinach and Tomato Omelets:

Cooking Time: 12 minutes

Serving: 1

Ingredients:

- 3 large eggs
- 1/2 cup fresh spinach, chopped.
- 1/4 cup cherry tomatoes, halved.

Instructions:

1. Whisk eggs in a bowl.
2. Pour eggs into a heated pan.
3. Add spinach and tomatoes, fold when cooked.

Nutritional Information: (per serving)

Calories: 230, Protein: 18g, Fat: 15g, Carbohydrates: 5g

Chia Seed Pudding with Berries:

Cooking Time: 5 minutes (plus chilling time)

Serving: 2

Ingredients:

- 1/4 cup chia seeds
- 1 cup lactose-free milk
- Mixed berries for topping

Instructions:

1. Mix chia seeds and milk, refrigerate for at least 4 hours or overnight.
2. Top with mixed berries before serving.

Nutritional Information: (per serving)

Calories: 180, Protein: 6g, Fat: 8g, Carbohydrates: 20g

Peanut Butter and Banana Rice Cakes:

Cooking Time: 5 minutes

Serving: 2

Ingredients:

- 2 rice cakes
- 2 tablespoons peanut butter
- 1 banana, sliced.

Instructions:

1. Spread peanut butter on rice cakes.
2. Top with banana slices.

Nutritional Information: (per serving)

Calories: 220, Protein: 6g, Fat: 10g, Carbohydrates: 30g

Blueberry Almond Smoothie Bowl:

Preparation Time: 10 minutes

Serving: 1

Ingredients:

- 1/2 cup blueberries
- 1/2 cup spinach
- 1/4 cup almonds
- 1 cup lactose-free yogurt

Instructions:

1. Blend blueberries, spinach, almonds, and yogurt until smooth.
2. Pour into a bowl and enjoy with additional toppings if desired.

Nutritional Information: (per serving)

Calories: 280, Protein: 15g, Fat: 15g, Carbohydrates: 25g

Turkey and Cheese Breakfast Wrap:

Cooking Time: 8 minutes

Serving: 1

Ingredients:

- 1 gluten-free wrap
- 2 slices low FODMAP deli turkey
- 1 slice Swiss cheese
- 1/2 cup spinach

Instructions:

1. Heat the wrap and add turkey and cheese.
2. Once the cheese is melted, add spinach.
3. Roll the wrap and serve.

Nutritional Information: (per serving)

Calories: 300, Protein: 20g, Fat: 15g, Carbohydrates: 20g

CHAPTER 3

LUNCHTIME FAVORITES

Grilled Chicken and Quinoa Salad:

Cooking Time: 20 minutes

Serving: 2

Ingredients:

- 2 boneless, skinless chicken breasts
- 1 cup cooked quinoa
- 1 cup cherry tomatoes, halved.
- 1 cup cucumber, diced.
- 1/4 cup feta cheese, crumbled.
- Olive oil, lemon juice, salt, and pepper for dressing

Instructions:

1. Grill chicken until fully cooked.
2. Slice chicken and combine with quinoa, tomatoes, cucumber, and feta.
3. Drizzle with olive oil and lemon juice, season with salt and pepper.

Nutritional Information: (per serving)

Calories: 400, Protein: 30g, Fat: 15g, Carbohydrates: 35g

Salmon and Asparagus Stir-Fry:

Cooking Time: 15 minutes

Serving: 2

Ingredients:

- 2 salmon fillets, cubed.
- 1 bunch asparagus, trimmed and cut into 2-inch pieces.
- 1 red bell pepper, sliced.
- 2 tablespoons low FODMAP stir-fry sauce

Instructions:

1. Stir-fry salmon until browned.
2. Add asparagus and bell pepper, stir in the sauce until vegetables are tender.

Nutritional Information: (per serving)

Calories: 350, Protein: 25g, Fat: 20g, Carbohydrates: 20g

Quinoa and Spinach Stuffed Bell Peppers:

Cooking Time: 30 minutes

Serving: 2

Ingredients:

- 1 cup cooked quinoa
- 2 cups fresh spinach, chopped.
- 2 bell peppers, halved.
- 1/2 cup feta cheese, crumbled.

Instructions:

1. Mix quinoa, spinach, and feta in a bowl.
2. Stuff the bell peppers with the mixture.
3. Bake until peppers are tender.

Nutritional Information: (per serving)

Calories: 300, Protein: 15g, Fat: 12g, Carbohydrates: 35g

Shrimp and Zucchini Noodles:

Cooking Time: 15 minutes

Serving: 2

Ingredients:

- 1 pound shrimp peeled and deveined.
- 2 zucchinis, spiralized
- 2 tablespoons garlic-infused olive oil
- Salt, pepper, and chopped parsley for seasoning

Instructions:

1. Sauté shrimp in garlic-infused olive oil until cooked.
2. Add zucchini noodles and cook until tender.
3. Season with salt, pepper, and parsley.

Nutritional Information: (per serving)

Calories: 250, Protein: 25g, Fat: 10g, Carbohydrates: 15g

Turkey and Quinoa Stuffed Tomatoes:

Cooking Time: 25 minutes

Serving: 2

Ingredients:

- 1 cup cooked quinoa
- 1/2-pound ground turkey
- 4 large tomatoes, hollowed.
- 1/4 cup chives, chopped.

Instructions:

1. Cook ground turkey until browned.
2. Mix quinoa, turkey, and chives, stuff into hollowed tomatoes.
3. Bake until tomatoes are soft.

Nutritional Information: (per serving)

Calories: 280, Protein: 20g, Fat: 10g, Carbohydrates: 30g

Eggplant and Tomato Stacks:

Cooking Time: 20 minutes

Serving: 2

Ingredients:

- 1 large eggplant, sliced.
- 2 large tomatoes, sliced.
- 1 cup mozzarella cheese, sliced.
- Fresh basil leaves

Instructions:

1. Grill eggplant slices until tender.
2. Assemble stacks with eggplant, tomato, and mozzarella.
3. Top with fresh basil.

Nutritional Information: (per serving)

Calories: 320, Protein: 15g, Fat: 15g, Carbohydrates: 25g

Chicken and Vegetable Skewers:

Cooking Time: 20 minutes

Serving: 2

Ingredients:

- 2 boneless, skinless chicken breasts, cubed.
- Zucchini, bell peppers, and cherry tomatoes, cut into chunks.
- Olive oil, lemon juice, salt, and pepper for marinade

Instructions:

1. Marinate chicken and vegetables in olive oil, lemon juice, salt, and pepper.
2. Thread onto skewers and grill until chicken is fully cooked.

Nutritional Information: (per serving)

Calories: 280, Protein: 25g, Fat: 12g, Carbohydrates: 20g

Tuna Salad Lettuce Wraps:

Preparation Time: 15 minutes

Serving: 2

Ingredients:

- 2 cans tuna, drained
- 1/4 cup mayonnaise
- 1 celery stalk finely chopped.
- Lettuce leaves for wrapping.

Instructions:

1. Mix tuna, mayonnaise, and celery in a bowl.
2. Spoon mixture onto lettuce leaves and wrap.

Nutritional Information: (per serving)

Calories: 250, Protein: 20g, Fat: 15g, Carbohydrates: 5g

Low FODMAP Sushi Bowl:

Cooking Time: 15 minutes

Serving: 2

Ingredients:

- 2 cups cooked sushi rice.
- 1/2-pound cooked shrimp, sliced.
- 1 cucumber, julienned
- 1 sheet nori, crumbled.
- Soy sauce (low FODMAP) for drizzling

Instructions:

1. Arrange rice, shrimp, cucumber, and nori in bowls.
2. Drizzle with low FODMAP soy sauce.

Nutritional Information: (per serving)

Calories: 300, Protein: 15g, Fat: 5g, Carbohydrates: 60g

Spinach and Feta Stuffed Chicken Breast:

Cooking Time: 30 minutes

Serving: 2

Ingredients:

- 2 boneless, skinless chicken breasts
- 1 cup fresh spinach, chopped.
- 1/4 cup feta cheese, crumbled.
- Olive oil, lemon juice, salt, and pepper for seasoning

Instructions:

1. Preheat oven to 375°F (190°C).
2. Mix spinach and feta, stuff into a pocket in each chicken breast.
3. Season with olive oil, lemon juice, salt, and pepper.
4. Bake until chicken is cooked through.

Nutritional Information: (per serving)

Calories: 320, Protein: 35g, Fat: 15g, Carbohydrates: 5g

CHAPTER 4

SATISFYING SNACKS

Greek Yogurt and Berry Parfait:

Preparation Time: 5 minutes

Serving: 1

Ingredients:

- 1 cup lactose-free Greek yogurt
- 1/2 cup strawberries, sliced
- 1/4 cup blueberries
- 1 tablespoon chia seeds

Instructions:

1. Layer yogurt, strawberries, blueberries, and chia seeds in a glass.
2. Repeat layers.
3. Top with a few extra berries.

Nutritional Information: (per serving)

Calories: 200, Protein: 15g, Fat: 8g, Carbohydrates: 20g

Hard-Boiled Eggs with Paprika:

Cooking Time: 12 minutes

Serving: 2

Ingredients:

- 4 hard-boiled eggs
- Paprika, salt, and pepper for seasoning

Instructions:

1. Peel hard-boiled eggs and cut in half.
2. Sprinkle with paprika, salt, and pepper.

Nutritional Information: (per serving)

Calories: 140, Protein: 12g, Fat: 9g, Carbohydrates: 1g

Rice Cake with Almond Butter and Banana:

Preparation Time: 5 minutes

Serving: 1

Ingredients:

- 1 rice cake
- 2 tablespoons almond butter
- 1/2 banana, sliced.

Instructions:

1. Spread almond butter on the rice cake.
2. Top with banana slices.

Nutritional Information: (per serving)

Calories: 220, Protein: 5g, Fat: 15g, Carbohydrates: 18g

Cucumber and Hummus Bites:

Preparation Time: 10 minutes

Serving: 2

Ingredients:

- 1 cucumber, sliced.
- 1/2 cup low FODMAP hummus
- Cherry tomatoes for topping

Instructions:

1. Spread hummus on cucumber slices.
2. Top with cherry tomatoes.

Nutritional Information: (per serving)

Calories: 150, Protein: 5g, Fat: 8g, Carbohydrates: 15g

Mixed Nuts and Seeds Trail Mix:

Preparation Time: 5 minutes

Serving: 1

Ingredients:

- 1/4 cup almonds
- 1/4 cup walnuts
- 1/4 cup pumpkin seeds
- 1/4 cup sunflower seeds

Instructions:

1. Mix almonds, walnuts, pumpkin seeds, and sunflower seeds in a bowl.

Nutritional Information: (per serving)

Calories: 300, Protein: 12g, Fat: 25g, Carbohydrates: 10g

Low FODMAP Caprese Skewers:

Preparation Time: 10 minutes

Serving: 2

Ingredients:

- Cherry tomatoes
- Fresh mozzarella balls
- Basil leaves
- Olive oil, balsamic vinegar, salt, and pepper for drizzling

Instructions:

2. Thread cherry tomatoes, mozzarella balls, and basil leaves onto skewers.
3. Drizzle with olive oil and balsamic vinegar, season with salt and pepper.

Nutritional Information: (per serving)

Calories: 180, Protein: 8g, Fat: 15g, Carbohydrates: 5g

Peanut Butter and Banana Smoothie:

Preparation Time: 5 minutes

Serving: 1

Ingredients:

- 1 ripe banana
- 2 tablespoons peanut butter
- 1 cup lactose-free milk

Instructions:

1. Blend banana, peanut butter, and milk until smooth.

Nutritional Information: (per serving)

Calories: 300, Protein: 10g, Fat: 18g, Carbohydrates: 30g

Roasted Chickpeas:

Preparation Time: 40 minutes

Serving: 2

Ingredients:

- 1 can (15 oz) chickpeas, drained and rinsed.
- 1 tablespoon olive oil
- 1 teaspoon paprika
- Salt and pepper to taste

Instructions:

2. Preheat oven to 400°F (200°C).
3. Toss chickpeas with olive oil, paprika, salt, and pepper.
4. Roast until crispy.

Nutritional Information: (per serving)

Calories: 220, Protein: 8g, Fat: 8g, Carbohydrates: 30g

Low FODMAP Salsa with Tortilla Chips:

Preparation Time: 15 minutes

Serving: 4

Ingredients:

- 2 cups tomatoes, diced.
- 1/2 cup green bell pepper, diced.
- 1/4 cup fresh cilantro, chopped.
- 1 tablespoon lime juice
- Tortilla chips (corn-based)

Instructions:

1. Mix tomatoes, bell pepper, cilantro, and lime juice in a bowl.
2. Serve with tortilla chips.

Nutritional Information: (per serving)

Calories: 120, Protein: 2g, Fat: 5g, Carbohydrates: 20g

Prosciutto-Wrapped Cantaloupe:

Preparation Time: 10 minutes

Serving: 2

Ingredients:

- 8 slices prosciutto
- 1/2 cantaloupe, cut into bite-sized pieces.

Instructions:

1. Wrap prosciutto slices around cantaloupe pieces.

Nutritional Information: (per serving)

Calories: 150, Protein: 10g, Fat: 8g, Carbohydrates: 10g

CHAPTER 5

DINNER DELICACIES

Grilled Lemon Garlic Chicken:

Cooking Time: 25 minutes

Serving: 2

Ingredients:

- 2 boneless, skinless chicken breasts
- 2 tablespoons garlic-infused olive oil
- Zest and juice of 1 lemon
- Salt, pepper, and fresh herbs for seasoning

Instructions:

2. Marinate chicken in garlic-infused olive oil, lemon zest, and juice.
3. Grill until fully cooked, seasoning with salt, pepper, and herbs.

Nutritional Information: (per serving)

Calories: 300, Protein: 30g, Fat: 15g, Carbohydrates: 5g

Low FODMAP Shrimp Stir-Fry:

Cooking Time: 20 minutes

Serving: 2

Ingredients:

- 1 pound shrimp peeled and deveined.
- Assorted low FODMAP vegetables (bell peppers, zucchini, carrots)
- 2 tablespoons garlic-infused olive oil
- Low FODMAP stir-fry sauce

Instructions:

1. Stir-fry shrimp and vegetables in garlic-infused olive oil.
2. Add low FODMAP stir-fry sauce until fully cooked.

Nutritional Information: (per serving)

Calories: 280, Protein: 25g, Fat: 12g, Carbohydrates: 15g

Quinoa Stuffed Bell Peppers with Turkey:

Cooking Time: 30 minutes

Serving: 2

Ingredients:

- 1 cup cooked quinoa
- 1/2-pound ground turkey
- 4 bell peppers, halved.
- 1 cup spinach, chopped.

Instructions:

1. Cook ground turkey until browned.
2. Mix quinoa, turkey, and spinach, stuff into bell peppers.
3. Bake until peppers are tender.

Nutritional Information: (per serving)

Calories: 320, Protein: 25g, Fat: 15g, Carbohydrates: 25g

Baked Salmon with Dill and Lemon:

Cooking Time: 20 minutes

Serving: 2

Ingredients:

- 2 salmon fillets
- 2 tablespoons fresh dill, chopped.
- Zest and juice of 1 lemon
- Salt and pepper to taste

Instructions:

1. Preheat oven to 400°F (200°C).
2. Place salmon on a baking sheet, season with dill, lemon zest, and juice.
3. Bake until salmon is cooked through.

Nutritional Information: (per serving)

Calories: 350, Protein: 30g, Fat: 20g, Carbohydrates: 5g

Eggplant and Zucchini Lasagna:

Cooking Time: 40 minutes

Serving: 4

Ingredients:

- 1 large eggplant thinly sliced.
- 2 zucchinis thinly sliced.
- 1 pound ground beef or turkey
- 2 cups low FODMAP marinara sauce
- 1 cup lactose-free mozzarella cheese, shredded.

Instructions:

1. Layer eggplant and zucchini slices in a baking dish.
2. Brown ground meat and layer over the vegetables.
3. Pour marinara sauce over and top with mozzarella.
4. Bake until bubbly and golden.

Nutritional Information: (per serving)

Calories: 400, Protein: 25g, Fat: 20g, Carbohydrates: 30g

Lemon Herb Baked Chicken Thighs:

Cooking Time: 35 minutes

Serving: 2

Ingredients:

- 4 bone-in, skin-on chicken thighs
- 2 tablespoons garlic-infused olive oil
- Zest and juice of 1 lemon
- Fresh herbs (rosemary, thyme) for seasoning

Instructions:

1. Preheat oven to 400°F (200°C).
2. Rub chicken thighs with garlic-infused olive oil, lemon zest, and juice.
3. Season with fresh herbs and bake until golden and crispy.

Nutritional Information: (per serving)

Calories: 350, Protein: 30g, Fat: 25g, Carbohydrates: 2g

Low FODMAP Quinoa and Vegetable Stir-Fry:

Cooking Time: 25 minutes

Serving: 2

Ingredients:

- 1 cup cooked quinoa
- Assorted low FODMAP vegetables (bell peppers, carrots, bok choy)
- 2 tablespoons sesame oil
- Low FODMAP soy sauce for seasoning

Instructions:

1. Stir-fry vegetables in sesame oil until tender.
2. Add cooked quinoa and season with low FODMAP soy sauce.

Nutritional Information: (per serving)

Calories: 300, Protein: 10g, Fat: 15g, Carbohydrates: 35g

Turkey and Spinach Stuffed Portobello Mushrooms:

Cooking Time: 30 minutes

Serving: 2

Ingredients:

- 4 large portobello mushrooms
- 1/2-pound ground turkey
- 2 cups fresh spinach, chopped.
- 1/4 cup feta cheese, crumbled.

Instructions:

1. Preheat oven to 375°F (190°C).
2. Remove mushroom stems and place on a baking sheet.
3. Brown ground turkey, mix with spinach and feta, stuff into mushrooms.
4. Bake until mushrooms are tender.

Nutritional Information: (per serving)

Calories: 320, Protein: 25g, Fat: 15g, Carbohydrates: 20g

Low FODMAP Lemon Herb Shrimp Skewers:

Cooking Time: 15 minutes

Serving: 2

Ingredients:

- 1 pound shrimp peeled and deveined.
- Zest and juice of 1 lemon
- Fresh herbs (parsley, dill) for seasoning
- Olive oil for drizzling

Instructions:

1. Thread shrimp onto skewers.
2. Mix lemon zest, juice, and herbs, drizzle over shrimp.
3. Grill until fully cooked.

Nutritional Information: (per serving)

Calories: 250, Protein: 20g, Fat: 15g, Carbohydrates: 5g

Low FODMAP Zucchini Noodles with Pesto:

Cooking Time: 15 minutes

Serving: 2

Ingredients:

- 2 large zucchinis, spiralized
- 1/2 cup homemade low FODMAP pesto
- Cherry tomatoes for garnish

Instructions:

1. Sauté zucchini noodles until tender.
2. Toss with low FODMAP pesto and garnish with cherry tomatoes.

Nutritional Information: (per serving)

Calories: 280, Protein: 8g, Fat: 25g, Carbohydrates: 10g

CHAPTER 6

SWEET TREATS

Low FODMAP Berry Smoothie Bowl:

Preparation Time: 10 minutes

Serving: 1

Ingredients:

- 1/2 cup strawberries
- 1/2 cup blueberries
- 1/2 cup lactose-free yogurt
- 1 tablespoon chia seeds

Instructions:

1. Blend strawberries, blueberries, and yogurt until smooth.
2. Pour into a bowl and top with chia seeds.

Nutritional Information: (per serving)

Calories: 200, Protein: 8g, Fat: 8g, Carbohydrates: 25g

Peanut Butter Banana Bites:

Preparation Time: 15 minutes

Serving: 2

Ingredients:

- 2 bananas, sliced.
- 2 tablespoons peanut butter
- 1/4 cup shredded coconut (unsweetened)

Instructions:

1. Spread peanut butter on banana slices.
2. Dip in shredded coconut.

Nutritional Information: (per serving)

Calories: 180, Protein: 4g, Fat: 10g, Carbohydrates: 20g

Low FODMAP Chocolate Dipped Strawberries:

Preparation Time: 20 minutes

Serving: 2

Ingredients:

- 1/2 cup dark chocolate chips (low FODMAP)
- 1 cup strawberries, washed and dried

Instructions:

1. Melt chocolate chips in a microwave-safe bowl.
2. Dip each strawberry in melted chocolate.
3. Place on parchment paper to cool.

Nutritional Information: (per serving)

Calories: 150, Protein: 2g, Fat: 10g, Carbohydrates: 15g

Almond Butter Energy Bites:

Preparation Time: 15 minutes

Serving: 12

Ingredients:

- 1 cup rolled oats.
- 1/2 cup almond butter
- 1/4 cup maple syrup
- 1/4 cup dark chocolate chips (low FODMAP)

Instructions:

1. Mix oats, almond butter, and maple syrup in a bowl.
2. Fold in chocolate chips.
3. Form into small energy bites and refrigerate.

Nutritional Information: (per serving - 2 bites)

Calories: 150, Protein: 4g, Fat: 8g, Carbohydrates: 15g

Low FODMAP Lemon Sorbet:

Preparation Time: 10 minutes

Freezing Time: 4 hours

Serving: 4

- Ingredients:
- 1 cup water
- 1/2 cup sugar
- Zest and juice of 2 lemons

Instructions:

1. Heat water and sugar in a saucepan until sugar dissolves.
2. Stir in lemon zest and juice.
3. Freeze in a shallow dish, scraping with a fork every hour.

Nutritional Information: (per serving)

Calories: 80, Protein: 0g, Fat: 0g, Carbohydrates: 20g

Coconut and Pineapple Popsicles:

Preparation Time: 10 minutes

Freezing Time: 4 hours

Serving: 4

Ingredients:

- 1 cup coconut milk
- 1 cup fresh pineapple, chopped
- 2 tablespoons shredded coconut (unsweetened)

Instructions:

1. Blend coconut milk and pineapple until smooth.
2. Stir in shredded coconut.
3. Pour into popsicle molds and freeze.

Nutritional Information: (per serving)

Calories: 120, Protein: 1g, Fat: 10g, Carbohydrates: 8g

Raspberry Almond Chia Pudding:

Preparation Time: 5 minutes (plus chilling time)

Serving: 2

Ingredients:

- 1/4 cup chia seeds
- 1 cup almond milk
- 1/2 cup raspberries
- 1 tablespoon sliced almonds

Instructions:

1. Mix chia seeds and almond milk, refrigerate for at least 4 hours or overnight.
2. Top with raspberries and sliced almonds before serving.

Nutritional Information: (per serving)

Calories: 150, Protein: 4g, Fat: 10g, Carbohydrates: 15g

Low FODMAP Banana Ice Cream:

Preparation Time: 5 minutes

Freezing Time: 2 hours

Serving: 2

Ingredients:

- 2 ripe bananas sliced and frozen.
- 1/4 cup lactose-free milk
- 1 teaspoon vanilla extract

Instructions:

1. Blend frozen banana slices, milk, and vanilla extract until smooth.
2. Freeze for an additional 2 hours.

Nutritional Information: (per serving)

Calories: 120, Protein: 1g, Fat: 0g, Carbohydrates: 30g

Maple Cinnamon Roasted Pecans:

Preparation Time: 15 minutes

Baking Time: 15 minutes

Serving: 4

Ingredients:

- 2 cups pecan halves
- 2 tablespoons maple syrup
- 1 teaspoon ground cinnamon
- Pinch of salt

Instructions:

1. Preheat oven to 325°F (163°C).
2. Toss pecans with maple syrup, cinnamon, and salt.
3. Bake until fragrant and toasted.

Nutritional Information: (per serving)

Calories: 250, Protein: 3g, Fat: 25g, Carbohydrates: 10g

Low FODMAP Chocolate Banana Oat Muffins:

Preparation Time: 15 minutes

Baking Time: 20 minutes

Serving: 6

Ingredients:

- 2 ripe bananas, mashed.
- 2 eggs
- 1 cup rolled oats.
- 1/4 cup cocoa powder (low FODMAP)
- 1/4 cup maple syrup
- 1 teaspoon baking powder

Instructions:

1. Preheat oven to 350°F (175°C).
2. Mix bananas, eggs, oats, cocoa powder, maple syrup, and baking powder.
3. Divide batter into muffin cups and bake until set.

Nutritional Information: (per serving - 1 muffin)

Calories: 150, Protein: 4g, Fat: 5g, Carbohydrates: 25g

CHAPTER 7

SPECIAL OCCASIONS

Grilled Salmon with Dill Sauce:

Cooking Time: 20 minutes

Serving: 4

Ingredients:

- 4 salmon fillets
- 2 tablespoons fresh dill, chopped
- 1 tablespoon olive oil
- **Salt and pepper to taste**

Instructions:

1. Preheat grill to medium-high heat.
2. Brush salmon with olive oil, sprinkle with dill, salt, and pepper.
3. Grill until salmon is cooked through.

Nutritional Information: (per serving)

Calories: 300, Protein: 25g, Fat: 18g, Carbohydrates: 2g

Low FODMAP Chicken Piccata:

Cooking Time: 30 minutes

Serving: 4

Ingredients:

- 4 boneless, skinless chicken breasts
- 1/4 cup lemon juice
- 1/2 cup chicken broth
- 2 tablespoons capers
- 2 tablespoons olive oil

Instructions:

1. Season chicken with salt and pepper, sauté in olive oil until golden.
2. Deglaze the pan with lemon juice and chicken broth.
3. Add capers and simmer until the sauce thickens.

Nutritional Information: (per serving)

Calories: 250, Protein: 30g, Fat: 12g, Carbohydrates: 4g

Herb-Crusted Rack of Lamb:

Cooking Time: 40 minutes

Serving: 2

Ingredients:

- 1 rack of lamb, trimmed.
- 2 tablespoons Dijon mustard
- 1/2 cup gluten-free breadcrumbs
- 2 tablespoons fresh rosemary, chopped.

Instructions:

1. Preheat oven to 400°F (200°C).
2. Rub lamb with Dijon mustard, coat with a mixture of breadcrumbs and rosemary.
3. Roast until the crust is golden and lamb is cooked to your liking.

Nutritional Information: (per serving)

Calories: 450, Protein: 25g, Fat: 35g, Carbohydrates: 10g

Quinoa and Roasted Vegetable Stuffed Bell Peppers:

Cooking Time: 40 minutes

Serving: 4

Ingredients:

- 2 cups cooked quinoa.
- Assorted low FODMAP roasted vegetables (zucchini, bell peppers, tomatoes)
- 1/4 cup pine nuts
- Fresh basil for garnish

Instructions:

1. Mix cooked quinoa with roasted vegetables and pine nuts.
2. Stuff bell peppers with the quinoa mixture.
3. Bake until peppers are tender.

Nutritional Information: (per serving)

Calories: 300, Protein: 8g, Fat: 10g, Carbohydrates: 40g

Shrimp and Avocado Salad with Lime Vinaigrette:

Preparation Time: 15 minutes

Serving: 2

Ingredients:

- 1 pound shrimp peeled and deveined.
- 2 avocados, diced.
- Mixed salad greens
- 2 tablespoons olive oil
- Juice of 1 lime

Instructions:

1. Sauté shrimp until cooked.
2. Toss shrimp with diced avocados and salad greens.
3. Whisk together olive oil and lime juice for the vinaigrette.

Nutritional Information: (per serving)

Calories: 350, Protein: 20g, Fat: 25g, Carbohydrates: 15g

Baked Lemon Herb Chicken Thighs:

Cooking Time: 35 minutes

Serving: 4

Ingredients:

- 8 bone-in, skin-on chicken thighs
- 2 tablespoons fresh parsley, chopped.
- Zest and juice of 2 lemons
- 1 tablespoon olive oil

Instructions:

1. Preheat oven to 375°F (190°C).
2. Rub chicken thighs with olive oil, lemon zest, and juice.
3. Bake until chicken is golden and cooked through.

Nutritional Information: (per serving)

Calories: 400, Protein: 30g, Fat: 30g, Carbohydrates: 2g

Low FODMAP Beef Tenderloin with Red Wine Reduction:

Cooking Time: 30 minutes

Serving: 2

Ingredients:

- 2 beef tenderloin steaks
- 1/2 cup red wine
- 1 tablespoon balsamic vinegar
- 1 tablespoon olive oil

Instructions:

1. Sear beef tenderloin steaks in olive oil until desired doneness.
2. Deglaze the pan with red wine and balsamic vinegar.
3. Simmer until the sauce thickens.

Nutritional Information: (per serving)

Calories: 450, Protein: 30g, Fat: 25g, Carbohydrates: 5g

Low FODMAP Lobster Tail with Garlic Butter:

Cooking Time: 20 minutes

Serving: 2

Ingredients:

- 2 lobster tails
- 1/2 cup unsalted butter
- 3 cloves garlic, minced.
- Fresh parsley for garnish

Instructions:

1. Split lobster tails in half and broil until cooked.
2. Melt butter in a pan, sauté minced garlic until fragrant.
3. Pour garlic butter over lobster tails, garnish with fresh parsley.

Nutritional Information: (per serving)

Calories: 350, Protein: 30g, Fat: 25g, Carbohydrates: 2g

Spinach and Feta Stuffed Chicken Roll-Ups:

Cooking Time: 40 minutes

Serving: 4

Ingredients:

- 4 chicken breasts pounded thin.
- 2 cups fresh spinach
- 1/2 cup feta cheese, crumbled.
- Olive oil, lemon juice, salt, and pepper for seasoning

Instructions:

1. Season chicken breasts with olive oil, lemon juice, salt, and pepper.
2. Layer with fresh spinach and crumbled feta, roll up and secure with toothpicks.
3. Bake until chicken is cooked through.

Nutritional Information: (per serving)

Calories: 300, Protein: 35g, Fat: 15g, Carbohydrates: 4g

Low FODMAP Chocolate Mousse:

Preparation Time: 20 minutes

Chilling Time: 2 hours

Serving: 4

Ingredients:

- 1 cup lactose-free dark chocolate
- 2 cups coconut cream
- 1 teaspoon vanilla extract
- 2 tablespoons maple syrup

Instructions:

1. Melt dark chocolate and let it cool.
2. Whip coconut cream until stiff peaks form.
3. Gently fold melted chocolate, vanilla extract, and maple syrup into the whipped cream.
4. Chill in the refrigerator for at least 2 hours before serving.

Nutritional Information: (per serving)

Calories: 400, Protein: 2, Fat: 35g, Carbohydrates: 20g

CHAPTER 8

14 DAY MEAL PLAN

Day 1:

1. Breakfast: Scrambled eggs with spinach and tomatoes.
2. Lunch: Grilled chicken salad with mixed greens, cucumber, and balsamic vinaigrette.
3. Dinner: Baked salmon with lemon and dill, quinoa, and steamed green beans.

Day 2:

1. Breakfast: Greek yogurt with strawberries and a sprinkle of chia seeds.
2. Lunch: Turkey and avocado lettuce wrap with a side of carrot sticks.
3. Dinner: Stir-fried shrimp with bell peppers and broccoli over a bed of rice.

Day 3:

1. Breakfast: Low FODMAP smoothie with banana, blueberries, lactose-free yogurt, and a handful of spinach.
2. Lunch: Quinoa salad with cherry tomatoes, cucumber, feta cheese, and a light olive oil dressing.
3. Dinner: Grilled chicken thighs with rosemary, roasted sweet potatoes, and sautéed zucchini.

Day 4:

1. Breakfast: Omelets with lactose-free cheese, bell peppers, and chives.
2. Lunch: Tuna salad with mixed greens, cherry tomatoes, and a side of grapes.
3. Dinner: Baked cod with a lemon and herb crust, steamed asparagus, and quinoa.

Day 5:

1. Breakfast: Overnight oats made with rolled oats, lactose-free milk, and topped with strawberries.
2. Lunch: Low FODMAP sushi rolls with tuna, avocado, and cucumber.
3. Dinner: Turkey and vegetable skewers with a side of grilled eggplant and a quinoa pilaf.

Day 6:

1. Breakfast: Smoothie bowl with kiwi, pineapple, and a sprinkle of gluten-free granola.
2. Lunch: Spinach and feta stuffed chicken breast, roasted carrots, and a side of green beans.
3. Dinner: Beef stir-fry with bok choy, bell peppers, and carrots served over rice.

Day 7:

1. Breakfast: Scrambled eggs with tomatoes and a side of orange slices.
2. Lunch: Low FODMAP chicken Caesar salad with romaine lettuce and cherry tomatoes.
3. Dinner: Grilled shrimp skewers with a side of quinoa and roasted Brussels sprouts.

Day 8:

1. Breakfast: Banana and peanut butter smoothie with lactose-free yogurt.
2. Lunch: Caprese salad with mozzarella, tomatoes, and fresh basil, drizzled with balsamic glaze.
3. Dinner: Baked chicken with a mustard and herb marinade, served with mashed potatoes and green beans.

Day 9:

1. Breakfast: Lactose-free yogurt parfait with strawberries and a handful of almonds.
2. Lunch: Turkey and cranberry wrap with lettuce and a side of sliced cucumber.
3. Dinner: Grilled swordfish with a lime and cilantro marinade, quinoa, and sautéed spinach.

Day 10:

1. Breakfast: Chia seed pudding made with lactose-free milk, topped with kiwi and raspberries.
2. Lunch: Shrimp and vegetable stir-fry with bok choy, bell peppers, and carrots, served with rice.
3. Dinner: Pork tenderloin with a maple and mustard glaze, sweet potato wedges, and steamed green beans.

Day 11:

1. Breakfast: Omelette with spinach, tomatoes, and lactose-free cheese.
2. Lunch: Low FODMAP Caesar salad with grilled chicken, romaine lettuce, and cherry tomatoes.
3. Dinner: Baked tilapia with a lemon and herb crust, quinoa, and roasted asparagus.

Day 12:

1. Breakfast: Smoothie with blueberries, banana, lactose-free yogurt, and a handful of spinach.
2. Lunch: Turkey and cranberry lettuce wraps with a side of carrot sticks.
3. Dinner: Grilled chicken skewers with a Mediterranean quinoa salad.

Day 13:

1. Breakfast: Greek yogurt with strawberries and a sprinkle of chia seeds.
2. Lunch: Low FODMAP sushi rolls with salmon, avocado, and cucumber.
3. Dinner: Beef and vegetable kebabs with a side of quinoa and roasted Brussels sprouts.

Day 14:

1. Breakfast: Overnight oats with rolled oats, lactose-free milk, and topped with raspberries.
2. Lunch: Spinach and feta stuffed chicken breast, roasted carrots, and a side of green beans.
3. Dinner: Baked cod with a lemon and herb crust, steamed asparagus, and quinoa.

CONCLUSION

As we reach the final pages of this Low FODMAP Diet Cookbook for Women, my heart swells with gratitude for the opportunity to be part of your culinary journey. The stories shared, the recipes savored, and the transformative power of healing through food have created a tapestry that extends far beyond these pages. It is my sincere hope that you, dear reader, have found not just a cookbook but a companion—a source of nourishment for both body and soul.

In the spirit of community and shared experiences, I encourage you to embark on this next phase of your culinary exploration with an open heart. Your feedback is not just welcomed; it is cherished. Share your triumphs and challenges, the moments of joy as well as those of reflection. Your insights can become the guiding stars for others navigating similar paths, creating a network of support that transcends the boundaries of these words.

As you close this cookbook and step into your kitchen, I invite you to consider the following:

- **Have you discovered a newfound appreciation for the connection between what you eat and how you feel?**
- **Are you eager to experiment with flavors, armed with the knowledge that each dish can be a step toward holistic well-being?**
- **In what ways has this cookbook transformed your relationship with food and, ultimately, your own body?**

Your journey does not end here; rather, it evolves into a tapestry woven with the threads of your unique experiences. Embrace the opportunity to share your story, for in doing so, you contribute to a collective narrative of strength, resilience, and the unwavering spirit of women supporting women.

Your feedback is not just a collection of words; it is a dialogue—an ongoing conversation that shapes the future editions of this cookbook and, more importantly, connects us in the shared pursuit of a vibrant and fulfilling life. Your insights have the power to inspire, guide, and uplift, creating a ripple effect that touches the lives of women who, like you, seek solace and nourishment.

As you embark on the culinary adventures inspired by these recipes, remember that your journey is as unique as your fingerprint. Embrace it with courage, savor each moment, and, above all, be kind to yourself. For in the gentle cadence of your kitchen, you are not just preparing meals; you are crafting a narrative of well-being and empowerment.

Thank you for inviting me into your culinary world, for allowing these recipes to become a part of your daily life. May the flavors linger on your palate, and the stories linger in your heart. And as you continue to explore the profound connection between food and well-being, may your experiences echo through the tapestry of shared stories, inspiring and uplifting the women who follow in your footsteps.

Please share your thoughts, your discoveries, and your own culinary creations. Your feedback is not just valuable; it is a celebration of the collective journey we embark upon together. Let your voice be heard, and let our community grow stronger with each shared experience.

With heartfelt gratitude and anticipation.

BONUS

MINDFUL EATING GUIDE

In the hustle and bustle of daily life, mealtime often becomes a rushed affair, with little attention paid to the sensory experience of eating. The Mindful Eating Guide within this cookbook is designed to reintroduce a sense of mindfulness into your culinary journey, emphasizing the significance of savoring each bite and reconnecting with your body's cues.

Key Practices:

Engage Your Senses:

Begin your mealtime ritual by taking a moment to appreciate the visual appeal, aromas, and textures of your food. Notice the vibrant colors, inhale the enticing scents, and run your fingers over the textures. Engaging your senses prepares your body for the nourishment it is about to receive.

Create a Tranquil Environment:

Whenever possible, set the stage for a peaceful and enjoyable dining experience. Dim the lights, play soft music, or choose a quiet space to eat. Minimize distractions such as phones or electronic devices to fully immerse yourself in the act of eating.

Chew Slowly and Thoroughly:

Mindful eating encourages you to savor each bite by chewing slowly and thoroughly. This not only aids in digestion but allows you to truly experience the flavors and textures of your food. Put your utensils down between bites and relish the taste lingering on your palate.

Acknowledge Hunger and Fullness:

Tune into your body's hunger and fullness cues. Before diving into your meal, assess your level of hunger. During the meal, periodically check in to identify the signals of fullness. This practice helps prevent overeating and fosters a healthier relationship with food.

Express Gratitude:

Take a moment to express gratitude for the nourishment before you. Whether it's a simple acknowledgment of the effort that went into preparing the meal or a reflection on the source of the ingredients, cultivating gratitude enhances the overall dining experience.

Mindful Portion Control:

Be mindful of portion sizes, serving yourself with the intention of providing your body with the sustenance it needs. Pay attention to feelings of satisfaction, allowing them to guide your decision to stop eating rather than relying on external cues.

Practice Intuitive Eating:

Intuitive eating involves listening to your body's signals and responding appropriately. Let go of external diet rules and trust your body's wisdom. This practice encourages a balanced approach to food and a more attuned connection with your body.

Reflect on Your Meal:

After finishing your meal, take a moment to reflect on the experience. How did the food make you feel? What flavors stood out to you? Reflecting on your meals fosters a deeper connection with your dietary choices and preferences.

Benefits of Mindful Eating:

Improved Digestion: Chewing food thoroughly aids in digestion and nutrient absorption.

Enhanced Satisfaction: Mindful eating promotes a sense of satisfaction, reducing the likelihood of overeating.

Better Food Choices: By paying attention to hunger and fullness cues, you are more likely to make balanced and nutritious food choices.

Stress Reduction: Creating a tranquil eating environment can contribute to stress reduction and a more enjoyable dining experience.